Your Body's Defenses

Your Body's Defenses

DAVID C. KNIGHT

McGRAW-HILL BOOK COMPANY
New York St. Louis San Francisco Montreal Toronto

The author wishes to thank Bernerd H. Burbank, M.D.
for reading the manuscript of this book.

Photographs on pages 11, 13, 53, 55 and 58
Courtesy of Culver Pictures, Inc.

Photographs on pages 51 and 60
Courtesy of the U.S. Department of Health, Education, and Welfare

Library of Congress Cataloging in Publication Data
Knight, David C
   Your body's defenses.
   SUMMARY: Describes the body's various natural
defenses against diseases and gives hints on how one can
reinforce these defenses with rest, proper nutrition, etc.
    1. Natural immunity—Juvenile literature.
[1. Natural immunity. 2. Hygien] I. Title.
RB153.K54   616.07'9   74-11083
ISBN 0-07-035105-8 (lib. bdg.)

123456789 BPBP 7898765

Contents

Your Body's Defenses

· 1 ·

Introduction

The "Wisdom of the Body"

We all know that miserable feeling when we wake up in the morning with a scratchy throat and realize that another cold is on the way. We all know the sharp pain—and the panic that follows—when we cut our finger deeply with a knife and the blood begins to flow. We have all experienced the gnawing dread as an unexpected boil grows alarmingly bigger and more painful. We are all familiar with that queasy, aching feeling when a powerful stomach virus seizes control of our digestive system and dooms us to a day or two of vomiting, diarrhea, and just plain misery.

Each one of us as a living human being has a body of flesh, blood, and bone. It is the only body we have. It must take us over a life span of many decades and through a world filled with hazards to our physical well-being. This system of flesh, blood, and bone— actually consisting of complex chemical compounds— possesses a remarkable set of defenses against attack from without—against accidents, injury, violence, and disease.

Our bodies—yours and mine—have an outer protective wall, many internal defenses, and a highly ingenious regulatory system. When we are attacked, somehow somewhere a chemical alarm goes off in our bodies, setting up a clangor to warn against invasion. Maybe the attacker is a virus; maybe bacteria. Whatever it is, something foreign and hostile has invaded our bodies, threatening their well-being. It is then that our bodies' protective mechanisms go to work, triggering highly complicated biochemical steps aimed at repelling the invader.

In addition, our bodies must often adjust to a changing environment in ways that are scarcely apparent to us. This adjustment is also a part of the body's system of defenses. For example, when we step outdoors on a bitterly cold day, all kinds of internal mechanisms are set in motion to neutralize the effects of the cold and keep the body on an even keel. To prevent body tem-

10

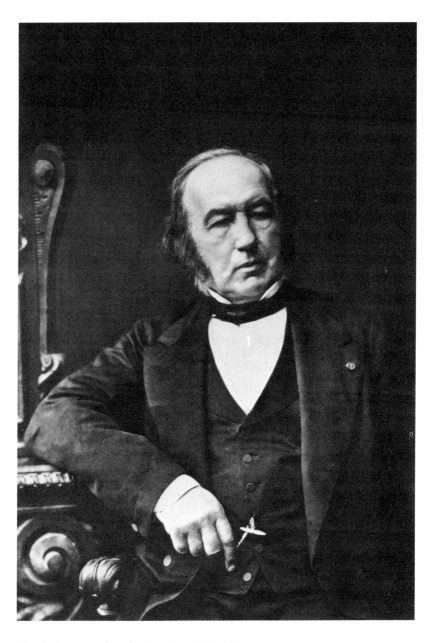

Claude Bernard, French physician, 1813–1878.

perature from dropping, the whole system undergoes certain changes designed to prevent heat loss through the skin. Nearly all perspiration stops. The blood vessels near the surface of the body constrict, slowing the flow of blood from the inner regions, so that less reaches the skin to become cooled.

The first man to focus scientific attention on these mechanisms was the French physician Claude Bernard, who died in 1878. Called today "the father of modern physiology," Bernard distinguished himself by applying the experimental method to his physiological research. At the same time that Charles Darwin was formulating his famous theory of evolution, Bernard was advancing equally important ideas in physiology, which he called "the science of the laws of life."

Charles Darwin's theory stated that only those individuals and species which are best fitted to their external environments survive. Dr. Bernard went one step further. He described this fitness as the ability to adapt to external changes while maintaining a constant *internal* environment. In this sense, fitness depends on the existence of control mechanisms which permit the body to maintain its individuality in the face of all challenges. Dr. Bernard put it this way: "The fixity of the internal environment is the essential requirement for a free life."

Later work in biochemistry proved Bernard right. It provided laboratory evidence that the chemical composition of the healthy body's tissues and fluids does remain constant within extremely narrow limits, regardless of external conditions. It also unraveled the chemical processes through which this constancy is

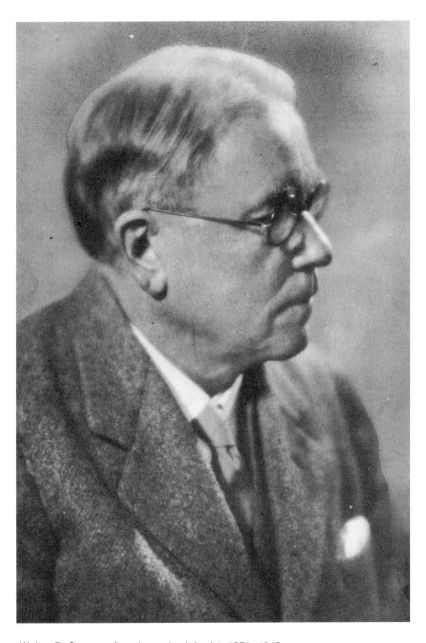

Walter B. Cannon, American physiologist, 1871–1945.

maintained. In the 1920s, the distinguished American physiologist, Walter B. Cannon, showed that these processes are chiefly controlled by the *autonomic* (involuntary) *nervous system* and by *hormones*, body chemicals that mediate the behavior of the various organs and organ systems.

Dr. Cannon was so impressed with the amazing efficiency of these body mechanisms that, when he wrote a book on the subject, he called it *The Wisdom of the Body*. In it, he coined a word generally used to describe the state produced by the constant adjustment a healthy body has to make. The word was *homeostasis*, a term from the Greek meaning "staying the same." It "does not imply something set and immobile," he wrote. "It means a condition—a condition which may vary, but which is relatively constant." Dr. Cannon went on to describe the complicated sequences by which the body maintains homeostasis with respect to such vital things as oxygen, water, salts, temperature, and blood pressure.

Of course, the body's "wisdom" has its limits, as Cannon very well knew. For one thing, the mechanisms for homeostasis do not come into being all at once. It takes some time before a newborn baby develops them. Before birth, the fluids and heat of the mother's body form an external environment that is virtually the same as that of the baby's own interior. It is only at birth that the infant comes into contact with surroundings that demand constant adjustments. At first, even a slight drop in the external temperature will produce a sharp drop in the baby's own temperature. But little by little, the infant develops the control mechanisms that

14

allow it to handle outside temperature changes quite easily.

When all the homeostatic mechanisms are working efficiently, every challenge the human body meets is handled in a way that prevents disease and permits continuous and healthy functioning.

Today, physiologists refer to the ability of the human body to react defensively against a foreign substance— whether it is a microorganism or some nonliving particle or molecule—as *immunity*. Immunity permits the person's body to destroy or neutralize the foreign substance more quickly than if it were not immune to it. The field of science that is concerned with the development of immunity and related biological processes is called *immunology*. Later, we shall examine this science and some of its progress.

Meanwhile, how do our bodies cope with the forces that would harm, invade, or destroy it? Let us look at our bodily defenses one by one, from the first lines of defense to the last.

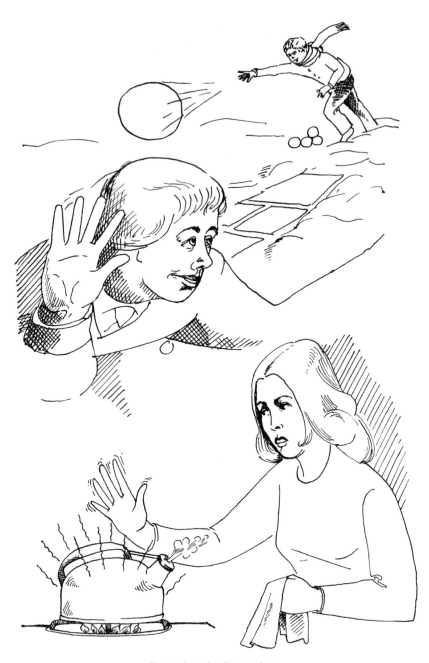

Examples of reflex actions.

16

·2·
The Body's Early Warning Apparatus
.
and Its Protective Responses

Even before danger threatens our bodies in a physical manner, we all have a built-in early warning system that tips us off—the human senses of sight, hearing, touch, taste, and smell. If we heed what our senses tell us, we can often avoid danger before it can harm us.

The organs of perception—our senses—warn us of

violence, due either to accident or to intentional attack by persons or animals. The eye can perceive or the ear detect the approach of something dangerous. For example, all of us have jumped out of the way of a fast-moving car that we just spied out of the corner of our eye. Or perhaps we did *not* see the car at all and a policeman's whistle warned us back to the curb in the nick of time.

While our sense of smell is less acute than that of many animals, it is still keen enough to warn us of the danger of injury from fire or smoke or attack. In addition, skin sensation—touch—is useful in detecting contacts with crawling insects, and other animals that may have a dangerous bite and in warning of excessive heat or cold. Touch also enables us to determine the texture of solid objects and the nature of fluids with which we may make contact. For example, if you accidentally put your hand in a bramble bush, your sense of touch tells you to withdraw it immediately before more damage is done. Even unpleasant tastes—say of spoiled food—warn us that further consumption of the substance will be sure to do us harm.

Our five senses are closely allied with the action of the body's nervous system. A warning signal received through the eye, the nose, the ear, or the skin is transmitted to the brain, which then takes appropriate action. If you have plenty of time, this may be a conscious action. In other words, you can think over what you want to do to avoid the danger. Say you are riding your bike down the street and you see a stalled car in the next block—right in your way. As you approach, you slow up and look the situation over, then decide

18

what to do next. But if there is an automobile directly ahead of you and the driver suddenly slams on his brakes, you do the same before you have a chance to size up the situation. This is called a *reflex action.*

A reflex action, or simply reflex, is a valuable line of defense against injury. It is an involuntary response. A reflex takes place when you duck without thinking when somebody throws a snowball at you. In fact, the chances are good you would duck even if you knew there was a heavy sheet of plexiglass between you and the oncoming snowball. Reflexes are also at work when you jerk your fingers away from a hot oven or range. Ex-combat soldiers have been known to "hit the dirt" instinctively when they hear a tire blowout. So similar is the noise to the explosion of an artillery shell that it triggers the reflex that saved their lives in wartime.

Here is a highly simplified description of how reflexes work. In the skin are tiny organs called *sensory receptors,* or simple receptors. They are located near the surface of the skin and are composed of sensitive cells or groups of cells. There is a different receptor for each sensation we feel—pain, cold, heat, pressure, surface texture, and so on. From these receptors, nerve fibers go through various nerve trunks to a nerve center, or *ganglion,* one of a chain which is just outside the backbone in the chest, abdomen, and neck, and in various places in the head. Here the impulse is delivered to other nerve fibers, much as a telephone relay carries the human voice from station to station, and the message is finally conveyed to the brain.

At this point, the stimulated brain initiates action impulses to cope with the specific situation. These

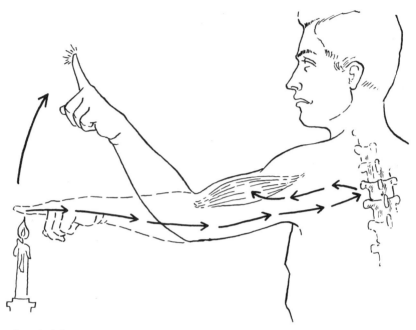

A part of the nervous system showing a reflex action.

impulses are transmitted to a nerve center in the spinal cord, and from there, by other connections, to muscles that bring the appropriate sense receptors—eyes, nose, fingers—into play. It is in this way that we look at, smell, or feel whatever stimulated our skin receptors.

If there is a real emergency, however, the whole process is short-circuited. Suppose your finger touches the runner of a sled left outdoors on an intensely cold day. You try to remove your finger and find out that it is sticking to the cold metal. A sensation of pain flashes to the spinal cord relay station. There it is intercepted and transmitted to the nerve fibers in the arm and hand

20

that bring about action. These fibers force the appropriate finger muscles to break the painfully cold contact instantly. This short-circuiting eliminates the extra time it would take for the danger signal to go through the brain.

Most of our reflexes serve a useful purpose. The blinking of the eye protects this organ from strong light and foreign bodies. The reflex withdrawal of an arm or a leg or finger from painful stimulation spares further injury. Action, such as walking, is aided by reflexes which alternately slow down and speed up movement of the leg muscles, thus coordinating their action. Reflexes increase the heartbeat and raise the blood pressure under conditions of stress and reverse these effects when the time of stress is over and the body is quiet. The sight, smell, or taste of food produces reflexes that stimulate the flow of digestive juices into the mouth, stomach, and intestines. And reflex activity is also involved in the acts of elimination, breathing, and even standing upright.

Another interesting reflex is the production of gooseflesh, the tiny bumps that appear on the body's skin during sudden cold. This reflex has little practical value today and probably dates back to the early days of the human race when men had a covering of thick hair. The goose bumps raised the hair on end, enclosing a protective layer of warmer air close to the body.

Actually, if the human body's resources fail to prevent a drop in temperature, two more reflex actions occur: the adrenal glands produce more adrenalin, and the person starts to shiver. Both result in increased muscle activity, which produces more heat in the body.

Many people believe that the sensation of pain is to be avoided at all costs. In reality, pain is one of the human body's most valuable safeguards. It is a signal that something is wrong and must be dealt with and remedied. Properly acted upon, pain is a safety device, a protective function of the body.

What exactly is pain? *Pain* is a feeling of discomfort arising from nerve endings in the skin tissue of the body. If you are hit with a baseball or get a splinter in your finger, you feel pain. But pain sensations can occur in many parts of the body other than the skin. For example, a headache can be brought on by a cold that irritates the sinuses or other pain-sensitive structures within the skull.

The kind of pain we feel varies with the particular part of the body involved. Moreover, pain can be steady or intermittent, sharp or dull, shooting or burning. If, for example, you pull a leg muscle, the pain is aching, likely to be spread in many directions up and down your leg, and it can come and go. Muscle pain can also be caused by the liberation of certain chemical substances into the tissues following vigorous exercise.

Bone pain is comparatively dull. Skin pain may be caused by intense heat, cold, or mechanical injury such as a cut or bruise. It can be either short-lived and sharp or long-lasting and burning. Intestinal pain may be produced by gas which stretches and twists pain-sensitive nerve endings.

When you have a toothache the pain is caused by fluid swellings within the bony canal of the tooth. This throbbing pain develops as your nerve endings are compressed with each beat of the pulse which drives blood

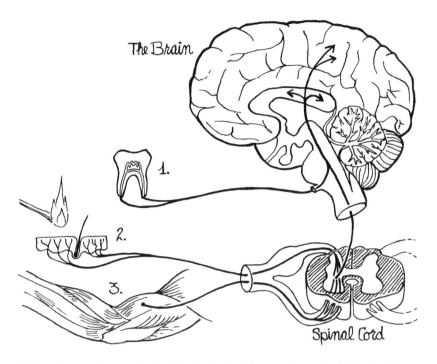

The Brain

1.

2.

3.

Spinal Cord

Various types of pain: 1. a toothache 2. heat 3. muscular pain. Pain signals go through nerves to the spine then to the brain.

into the inflamed and swollen canal. Whatever the pain, it is one of the body's best sentinels for it serves the all-important purpose of indicating that something is wrong and must be put right again.

Closely related to pain are other uncomfortable sensations such as dizziness, itching, faintness, and nausea. For example, if you occasionally feel faint, this sensation may mean that iron or some other important nutrient is lacking in your diet. Or, if you have been troubled by some itchy red patches on one of your arms, you may have a skin ailment called psoriasis. Like pain, these discomforts indicate to us that some bodily func-

23

tion is out of kilter and needs attention. They should be heeded well, particularly if they are severe, if they tend to recur at frequent intervals, and if they persist for more than a few hours.

Fever is also part of your body's early warning apparatus. *Fever* is an abnormal elevation of body temperature that usually occurs in response to an invasion of the body by germs. The average healthy body temperature, 98.6 degrees Fahrenheit, is maintained by an accurate balance between heat production and heat loss. The body's production of heat is increased by exercise, shivering, and contraction of the muscles. The digestion of food and certain types of glandular activity also contribute to heating the body. Heat is lost by sweating, by vaporization of water from the lungs, and by ordinary radiation of heat away from the body's surface.

When a fever breaks out, the person perspires heavily so that heat loss exceeds heat production and the temperature returns to normal. Fever can also occur without infection, as in cases of heat stroke in which there is a disturbance of the heat-regulating mechanism, as in injury to the brain which damages the heat-regulating center, or after the injection of foreign proteins into the body.

·3·
The First Line of Defense Against Infection
·
the Skin and Mucous Membranes

Diseases that attack the human body from without are met with what military commanders would call defense-in-depth; that is, when one defense is broken through, another stands ready to take over. The skin is the natural barrier to disease germs and is, together with the mucous membranes, the body's first line of defense.

25

Both the skin and mucous membranes of your body are, of course, composed of *cells.* All living things are made of cells. Most are so small that they can be seen only under a microscope. The human body has many kinds of cells. Each has its special job, special shape, and special place. Cells of one kind are usually joined together to make tissue. (Blood cells are an exception; they are not joined but travel alone.) A *tissue* is actually a living fabric woven of the same kind of cells. For example, muscles are tissue made of muscle cells; nerves are tissue made of nerve cells; and skin and mucous membrane are tissue formed of skin and mucous membrane cells.

Your body's skin is a remarkable first line of defense in many ways. It is waterproof and germproof when it remains unbroken. Attacking germs cannot really get inside the body until they have successfully penetrated the skin that covers it or the mucous membranes that line it. The digestive and respiratory systems, commonly considered to be inside us, are really outside the body proper; they are covered with mucous membrane that resists penetration. Thus, healthy tissues in the mouth, alimentary canal, and natural body openings resist infection as well as healthy skin tissue such as that which covers our arms and legs.

The mucous membranes afford protection through the chemical compositions they secrete. The slightly acid saliva in the mouth and the more strongly acid stomach secretions both help keep germs to a healthy minimum. The salty fluid called tears produced in the eyes also kills germs. In the nose, the membranes have tiny *cilia,* or hairlike structures, which wave rhythmically, moving out secretions, dust, germs, and other foreign material. Incidentally, the sudden exhalation of breath we call sneezing, caused by irritation of the mucous membranes, serves to clear the nasal passages of unwanted material.

In reality, the skin is a double line of defense because it consists of two layers. The upper, or outer, layer is called the *epidermis*. Beneath it is the layer called the *dermis*, or "true skin." Let us examine each briefly to see how the skin as a whole performs so well as a defender of our bodies.

The outer layer, or epidermis, is thickest on the soles of the feet and the palms of the hands. It is relatively

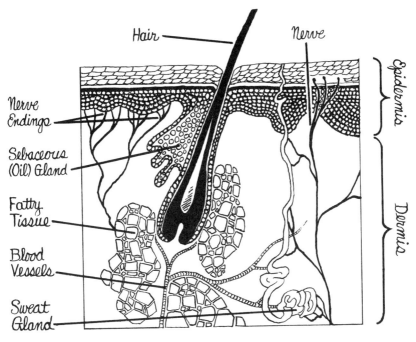

A cross-section of the skin showing the epidermis and dermis.

thin on the rest of the body. The epidermis is marked by numerous elevated ridges that correspond to ridges in the underlying true skin. These outer ridges increase friction between the skin and contact surfaces when a person is walking or grasping objects. Moreover, the pattern of ridges on the fingertips is unique to each person, a fact that makes fingerprints a valuable means of identification.

When you go swimming, you have probably noticed that your skin sheds water. If the skin absorbed water, our bodies would soon become waterlogged; swimming, showering, and bathing would be difficult. The reason the epidermis sheds water is that it is normally covered by a water-resistant, oily, fatty secretion from the sebaceous glands and contains a water-insoluble protein called keratin.

If you play a lot of tennis, you probably have some calluses on your racket hand. Or if you have done some heavy jogging or cross-country hiking lately, the chances are you have a corn or two to show for it. Corns and calluses are outgrowths of the epidermis and are caused by mechanical irritation of the skin. They are a protective thickening of the outer skin layer and serve to shield the more delicate tissues underneath.

The coloring of the skin depends in part on the pigment called *melanin* contained in the epidermis. The color of the skin is basically yellow, but a reddish tint is contributed by the blood vessels of the dermis and a brownish cast is added by the pigment particles of the epidermis. The epidermis of darker-skinned people contains greater quantities of melanin. Sunlight stimulates the formation of melanin in the skin, an effect we recognize as tanning.

One of the chief defenses of the epidermis is actually caused by the daily wear and tear it undergoes. A natural barrier is provided by the outer layers of dead, flattened cells, which flake or slough off without damage to the body and without pain. You can see this happen in the summertime when the dead skin of your suntan peels. Also, after you take a bath, the residue you see in the tub is not so much dirt as it is dead skin. These dead skin cells are constantly being replaced by new growth in the underlying layer of the epidermis. The epidermis itself has no blood supply of its own but is nourished by nutrients supplied by the blood vessels of the dermis.

The dermis, or true skin, contains sweat glands, hair roots, the sebaceous glands (which provide the epidermis with its waterproof oiliness), nerves, and blood vessels suspended in a network of tough connective tissue fibers. It is the blood vessels of the dermis which rush blood to any menaced area of the skin and thus bring to bear forces that fight invading germs.

We sweat, or perspire, through the simple, coiled tubular sweat glands of the dermis. The evaporation of sweat from the skin serves to cool the body and is one of the principal means of temperature regulation. At moderate temperatures, the sweat evaporates immediately and we do not feel it. But at higher temperatures, particularly when the air is humid, the sweat collects on the skin and we feel the discomfort so familiar on hot, humid days. The summer complaint of prickly heat is caused by the blockage of the sweat glands. When we sweat excessively, salt is lost in perspiration and the electrochemical balance of the body may be upset, causing muscle cramps.

The flow of blood to our skin serves two important purposes: it nourishes the skin and it regulates the temperature of the body. Blood loses heat as it passes through the vessels of the skin. This flow of blood to the skin is regulated by the opening or closing of the blood vessels. This action is made possible by nerves that end on the smooth muscle walls of small vessels in the skin. The nerves belong to the vast network of the nervous system that unconsciously coordinates the activity of the heart, glands, and other internal organs. Warming of the body causes reflex expansion of the blood vessels, bringing more blood to the skin to be cooled. Similarly, when the body is overly cool, the blood vessels constrict, thus reducing the flow of blood and heat loss through the skin.

Below the dermis is yet another natural barrier that serves to protect us. This is the layer of subcutaneous tissue, or fat. (*Subcutaneous* means "under the skin.") This fatty layer protects the body by storing up valuable heat and also by serving as a cushion against blows and falls.

·4·
When the Body Is Invaded
·
Antigens on the Attack

All of us have at some time been troubled by slight infections. Perhaps a splinter became lodged under your fingernail and, for a day or two as it worked itself out, you felt a painful throbbing sensation. Or, after a day of swimming at the seashore, you may have neglected a shell cut that in time began to fester and swell. Certainly no such minor infection, however slight, should be ignored; for our own safety we should seek medication and proper treatment at the earliest opportunity.

If the skin of our body is broken, the way is prepared for infection to enter. Small cuts or breaks heal quickly, first being sealed against invasion by the clotted blood, which not only prevents *hemorrhage* (excessive blood loss) but also constitutes a defense against infection by germs. If, however, infection has been introduced at the time of injury, there may be a smaller center of inflammation around the affected area. It will turn reddish and there will be pain or throbbing and heat. Perhaps *abscesses*—collections of pus—will form. A typical abscess on the surface of the body is a hard, painful lump or swelling known as a *boil.*

Briefly, here is what happens when the infection sets in. Additional blood is rushed to the skin-break area, which accounts for the increase in temperature in that area, and the blood brings with it more white cells— one of the body's main defenses against germs. The biological name for these white cells which swallow up unwanted things is *phagocytes* from the Greek words meaning "eating cells." There is more than one kind of white cell. Some circulate in the blood while others wander or remain fixed in the tissues and other parts of the body. If germs get into the body through a cut in the skin, little blood phagocytes called *polymorphonuclear cells* engulf them. Then large phagocytes called *monocytes* assemble. These swallow up any dead cells and debris as well as any remaining bacteria.

When infection sets in, the white blood cells do not remain inside the blood vessels or the smaller hairlike

32

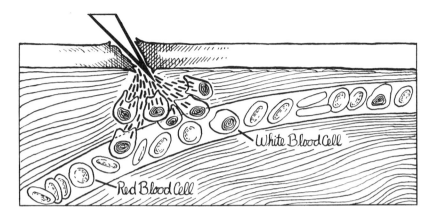

A break in the skin. Germs enter, but white cells attack them.

vessels called *capillaries*. Rather, they ooze through the thin and easily permeated vessel walls into the surrounding tissues. There they meet any invading organisms and try to surround and destroy them. In so doing, the accumulations of pus called abscesses may form. *Pus* is the fluid that gathers in abscesses as a reaction to inflammation caused by germs. It consists

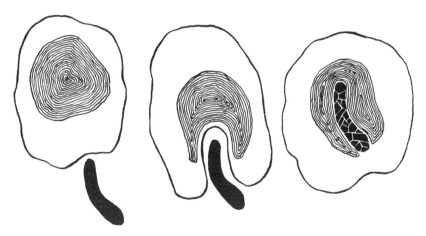

White cells (phagocytes) attacking and capturing germs.

mainly of white blood cells, dead tissue cells, and living or dead germs. Pus may be thin and watery or thick and jellylike, and either greenish white or yellowish, depending on the germs that caused the inflammation.

The inflammation process is the response of tissue cells when they are hurt. The injury may come from a blow, a burn, a cut, or chemical or radiation damage. In repairing the damage, the body musters a whole chain of reactions. The injured part becomes red, fevered, swollen, and sore, indicating that the white cells have already arrived on the scene.

If you could see a cross section of an abscess in its early inflammatory stages, you would see tissues swollen with blood which make a protective wall around the entry area of the infection. If the infection is successfully held in check, the center of the abscess liquefies and the outcome of the battle is pus. The invading bac-

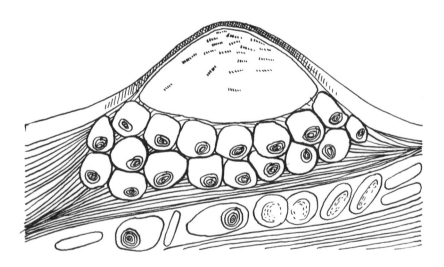

A boil showing swollen tissue, forming a wall and white cells.

teria lie at the center of the abscess, surrounded by the defending white blood cells. At this stage, we commonly say that the abscess "comes to a head," or "points." Then it is ready to be opened; that is, lanced or drained. The pus that is discharged contains white blood cells with their engulfed bacteria, dead tissues from the site of the abscess, and bacterial poisons. If an abscess or a boil is lanced too soon, the protective wall of blood-swollen tissues may become punctured and the microbial invaders can escape, causing infection to spread to healthy surrounding tissues or even into the bloodstream.

The same thing can happen in the case of a seemingly innocent-looking pimple. Pimples are the familiar skin eruptions we all experience occasionally. They are similar to abscesses but smaller. When you squeeze a pimple, you may be letting yourself in for some harmful consequences. The squeezing may force the infected material into surrounding healthy tissues and cause them to become infected, too. The wisest way to deal with pimples is not to squeeze or attempt to drain them at all. As with some abscesses, they may not *need* to be opened. If the white blood cells have succeeded in destroying the infectious germs, the pus is absorbed into the body and the abscess, boil, or pimple vanishes. The safest course in dealing with abscesses, boils, or persistent pimples which appear to need draining is to consult a doctor or, at least, a knowledgeable adult.

In a very real sense, the invasion of our bodies by infectious germs can be likened to war. At the points of attack, there are local skirmishes, followed later by full-fledged battles. In this "war," the cells and the

35

chemical consituents of the blood, tissue cells, and body fluids represent the defending forces against the invaders. The phagocytes can be compared to the infantry, which does the fighting and which mops up after the battle. Either the enemy is repelled or the defenders are overwhelmed.

The body is quick to recognize foreign chemicals that enter it. The "foes" must be attacked or otherwise gotten rid of. The most common of these foes are chemical materials from harmful bacteria, viruses, molds, and other microscopic organisms. Such invading chemicals, when recognized by the body, are called *antigens*. Antigens may enter the body through a cut or be breathed in or swallowed. To better understand the nature of antigens and how the body repels them, let us look at some of the microorganisms that can serve as antigens.

Microorganisms, or *microbes*, are tiny living things that can be seen only with a microscope. Most microbes are harmless. Some are even useful, but others are very harmful to human beings. Those that cause diseases are called germs. Microbes are of four main types: bacteria, molds and yeasts, protozoa, and viruses.

Bacteria are tiny one-celled plants; their types are grouped according to shape. A ball-shaped type is called a coccus. An oblong or rod-shaped form is called a bacillus. A curved type is known as a spirillum. Bacteria are very small—1/10,000 to 1/50,000 of an inch in diameter.

Bacteria feed on other plants and on animals. Each kind of bacterium lives and multiplies only where it gets the food it needs. For example, the bacteria that

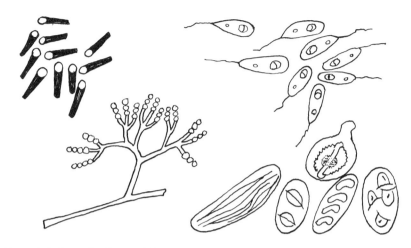

Upper left: bacteria, Upper right: protozoa, Lower left: mold, Lower right: yeasts. Not to scale.

cause tuberculosis live only in animal tissues such as lungs or in animal products such as milk. Bacteria multiply by dividing into two parts. Each part grows to maturity and then again splits in two. With the proper food supply and other necessary conditions, one cell could theoretically multiply with fantastic speed and produce in about three days a mass of bacteria weighing 7,000 tons. Fortunately, this does not actually occur because the growth of bacteria is checked when their food supply is used up, or their own waste material halts their growth. Also, man has learned many ways of checking the growth and reproduction of harmful bacteria.

In order to live and multiply, most bacteria need moisture, proper temperature (usually warm), food, oxygen, protection from ultraviolet light, and an absence of acids and strong chemicals. Bacteria and other germs outside the body can, therefore, be killed or prevented from growing by removing one of these essentials.

If the body is successfully invaded by harmful microbes and these germs increase to great numbers, they give off poisons called *toxins*, which can serve as antigens. These toxins in a person's blood make him ill. The symptoms usually include headache, nausea, and fever. Often a rash appears.

Most *molds* are harmless, threadlike plants which grow on food such as cheese and bread. Some molds, however, can grow on human skin and cause diseases, for example, ringworm, athlete's foot, and barber's itch.

Yeasts are single-celled plants that reproduce by a process called budding. Little growths or projections grow on an adult plant, break off, and then grow to maturity themselves. Most yeasts are harmless; some are used in making beer, bread, cake, and wine. But a few yeasts and yeastlike organisms can cause serious ulcers and lesions (injuries) to the skin, bone, and lungs of human beings.

Protozoa are tiny one-celled animals. Very few of them cause human disease. Yet some are very harmful. An example is the protozoan that causes malaria. This germ passes part of its life in the body of a human being (or other animal such as a cow or horse) and part of its life in the body of an insect (the anopheles mosquito). A person can get malaria only when bitten by an anopheles mosquito that has these malaria protozoa in its body.

African sleeping sickness is another dangerous disease that is caused by a different kind of protozoan, one which lives part of its life in the body of a human being and part in the body of the tsetse fly. Amebic dysentery is a very serious disease caused by a protozoan called an ameba. This protozoan lives in the human intestines. In tropical countries where the sanitation is bad, it is not safe to eat raw vegetables because they may be contaminated by these dangerous amebas. With bad sanitation, the human wastes from those who have this disease contaminate the soil.

Viruses are usually much smaller than bacteria. Most of them are too small to be seen with an ordinary microscope. As yet, scientists know comparatively little about the viruses and their many strains. It is known that the blood or waste matter of animals sick with a virus disease can transmit the same disease to others. Scientists believe that some of the commonest of human diseases—colds, influenza, measles, smallpox, yellow fever, rabies, and infantile paralysis—are caused by various types of viruses. Although virus-caused diseases have been very difficult to control, scientists are at work night and day in an effort to track down and limit these germs which cause so much human discomfort and misery.

These, then, are the various forms of invading antigens that attack our bodies. In addition to the defense provided by white cells, what can our bodies do to defeat them?

·5·

The Main Line of Defense

·

Antibodies to the Rescue

Against the attack by antigens our bodies have an ingenious chemical defense. Indeed, it is the body's main line of defense in combating the forces that would take over and destroy it.

The invaded tissues soon begin producing their own chemicals called *antibodies*, protein molecules which counteract the effects of hostile microbes. There are

40

several kinds of antibodies, and each invading antigen causes a specific kind of antibody to be produced.

After the antigens have entered the body, antibodies begin to form within a few days. They reach their greatest numbers after two weeks or so. When the threat is gone, some of the antibodies remain in the blood. If a sick person gets well without the aid of drugs or medicine, it is because his body has produced enough of these antibodies to overcome the germs and their toxins. Even when a doctor prescribes medicine, he still expects a person's production of antibodies to participate in combating the offending antigens.

Antibodies are also important when certain diseases threaten the body again. The body makes more antibodies within a day or two. This is what happens, for example, with smallpox or measles. One attack enables a person to make enough antibodies to repel the disease a second time if he becomes reinfected.

What is the structure of antibodies? The molecules of antibodies, like those of typical antigens, are very large. Scientists now think that most of them are cigar-shaped. Antibodies are of course made of protein; next to water, protein is the main stuff of the body and its cells.

Like other proteins, antibodies consist of long chains of smaller units called *amino acids*. These are the protein building blocks, and there are about twenty different kinds of them. A typical protein chain may contain several hundred amino acid units. These units occur one after another in a definite pattern. It is this pattern that determines the protein itself.

Once this antibody pattern is made, the protein chain

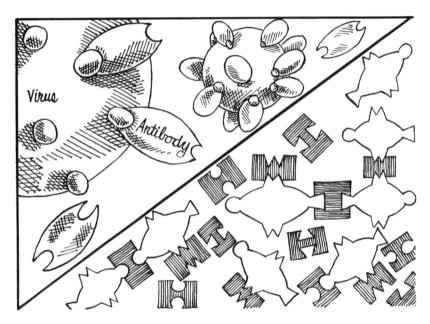

Antibodies attack viruses by fitting over them. There are two ways they might do it.

takes on a "second-order structure," often a spiral or a helix. Next, this spiral folds in on itself in an intricate way so that each protein molecule has a complex three-dimensional shape. It is this "third-order structure," as scientists call it, that permits it to carry out its specific job, as we shall see.

All antibodies belong to a group of proteins called *globulins*. The most common globulins are found in the blood and are called *gamma globulins*. Although they are big, their chemically active areas are known to be small. So are those of the antigen molecules. There are probably not more than two or three of these active areas on each gamma globulin molecule, taking up perhaps one percent of its entire surface. The general

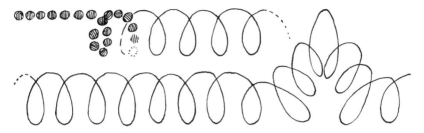
Antibodies showing second and third order structures.

chemical term for all antibodies is *immunoglobulin*, abbreviated Ig.

Scientists have two leading theories about how antibodies are formed in order to carry out their defensive jobs: the instruction theory and the selection theory. In the instruction theory, the shape of the antigen's active area determines what the shape of its antibody will be; that is, it "instructs" or dictates the antibody's configuration. As the invading antigen makes its way into a

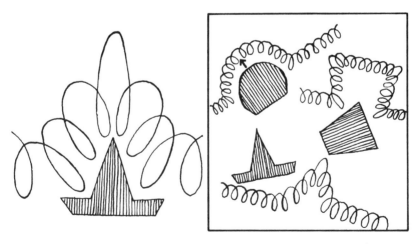
A diagram showing instruction and selection theories as to how antibodies attack antigens.

cell, a globulin molecule makes contact with it. This occurs just as the globulin is folding into its third-order structure. In this way, the antigen acts as a mold, or template, for the enfolding antibody. According to this theory, the active areas of the antigen fit into the newly molded pockets of the antibody the way a key fits into a lock or a lead soldier fits into its mold.

In the selection theory, a certain cell or group of cells instinctively "knows"—selects—how to make an antibody for a particular antigen. This can be done for thousands of possible antigens because the particular cell or cell family carries inherited information in its nucleus for making that specific antibody. When an antigen invades the body, it stimulates the cells to make the right antibody to react against it.

Where do antibodies come from? Scientists now think that they are made by certain kinds of white cells called *plasma cells*. In turn, they believe that the plasma cells themselves come from other white cells in the body called *lymphocytes*. In any case, antibodies are manufactured in organs that have large numbers of lymphocytes. Chief among these lymphoid areas are the lymph nodes and the spleen, both of which are important antibody "factories." After antibodies are formed in these lymphoid organs, they enter the bloodstream and are circulated throughout the body. Thus, antibodies made in a lymph node in a person's armpit against a certain antigen can prevent the growth and spread of like antigens that enter, say, a scratch in the leg.

Many antigens are too large to stimulate lymphocytes directly. These antigens have to be broken down

44

into smaller bits before they bring about the production of antibodies. This process is done by special white blood cells called *macrophages* (literally, "big eaters"). These cells, like the smaller lymphocytes, are present in lymphoid tissues.

What happens if the body loses the local skirmish and the defending antibodies are overwhelmed by invading antigens? Fortunately, the body has another line of defense—the lymph nodes themselves. Part of the tissue fluids drain through a series of vessels that parallel the veins and eventually convey these fluids (called lymph) into two large veins. These vessels lead through collections of spongy tissue known as *lymph nodes*; they constitute strainer-like traps for infectious germs.

The lymph nodes are strategically placed at circulation "bottlenecks," which might correspond to easily defended outposts, such as mountain passes, where an alert military commander would station his reserve forces. Widely distributed throughout the body, most lymph nodes are less than one-half an inch long. You can probably feel some of the larger ones under the skin in your armpit, in the groin, or in your neck just under the jaw. Others are located near the elbow and the knee.

Within the lymph nodes, the invading antigens are attacked by lymphocytes. These trap the antigens by engulfing them and eventually removing them from the bloodstream. During periods of active antibody production, the lymph nodes often swell considerably and may be tender to the touch. This is why sore lumps may develop in the armpit after a vaccination in the arm and why the groin nodes may swell up after a boil

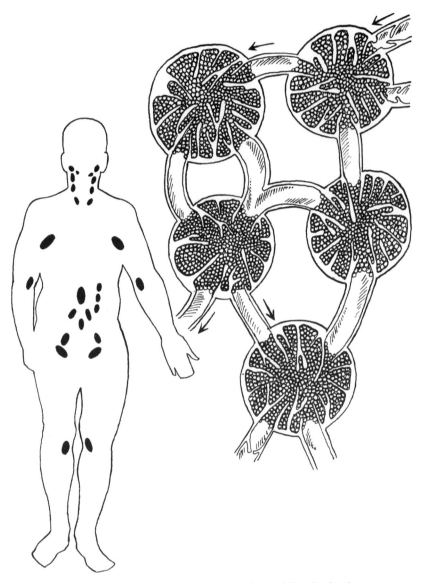

The location of the lymph glands and enlarged views of lymph glands.

forms on the leg. Sometimes the lymph nodes temporarily break down in the process of handling heavy infections and form abscesses; however, they still perform their job of protecting the main body structure and the vital organs.

An infection that has overcome the body's local defenses can often be traced by angry red lines running from the point of injury up the arm or leg. These lines are the inflamed lymph vessels, which are draining away the fluids containing the infectious microbes. There are also systems of lymph nodes and drainage vessels that serve the internal organs in the same manner as the superficial nodes serve the arms and legs.

·6·

The Science of Immunology

.

The Many Reactions of the Body to Disease

Immunology is the scientific study of how our bodies resist invasions by outside organisms or substances. As we know, these invaders are called antigens and they may be bacteria, viruses, protozoa, or other harmful microbes. The way your body reacts to a blood transfusion or a transplanted organ such as a kidney is also the concern of immunology.

In reacting to these things, certain groups of the

48

body's cells must make a kind of chemical choice. They accept what belongs to the body and reject intruders which do not belong. Getting rid of the intruders, or attempting to, is called an *immune response.*

The body has a wide range of immune responses, as we have seen previously. Generally they are useful and protect our bodies from disease. But sometimes these same responses are overactive. Allergies and some other serious disorders appear to be nothing more than confused immune responses. Likewise, in so-called "spare parts" surgery, the body may wholly reject a transfusion, a skin graft, or a transplanted heart or kidney.

As a result, medical scientists are doing a great deal of research work to find out more about immune responses. These responses of the body are often divided into two kinds: native immunity and acquired immunity.

Native immunity is the resistance that the body has inherited to many different organisms. For example, human beings simply do not catch dog distemper; nor does a dog ever come down with a human cold.

Within the same species, certain individuals are far more resistant than others to certain diseases. For example, the tuberculosis bacillus is found practically everywhere. Yet not every person contracts the disease of tuberculosis when exposed to it. At present, scientists still do not know a great deal about why these differences in native immunity exist. But in general, a person's native resistance to disease depends on the body's skin barriers, chemical agents, inflammatory process, and other defenses already discussed.

Acquired immunity is resistance to an organism that a person develops himself. While native immunity gives general protection against most invaders, acquired immunity protects against only one kind of antigen. Acquired immunity depends on the body's ability to make antibodies. The body's own experience with an antigen leads it to produce an antibody that reacts to that particular antigen and probably to no other.

Physicians take advantage of their knowledge of acquired immunity to protect people against diseases. They know that killed or altered antigens, when injected into a person, can cause antibodies to be produced. The antibodies then combat the disease that the antigen causes, and the person is thus protected against the disease. Such acquired immunity is man-made and is sometimes called *artificial immunity*.

Antigens prepared and injected in this fashion are called *vaccines*. Since the vaccinated person (or animal) has to make his own antibodies rather than get them from someone else, the procedure is referred to as *active immunization*. Injecting an antigen to start the production of antibodies is called *vaccination*.

Active immunization is commonly used to protect people from such diseases as cholera, typhus, typhoid fever, smallpox, yellow fever, measles, diphtheria, whooping cough, tetanus, and rabies, as well as poliomyelitis. A series of injections, or shots, may be required to deal with these diseases. Later, the person may need a booster shot, which raises the number of antibodies in his body.

Antibodies may be taken from one person and given

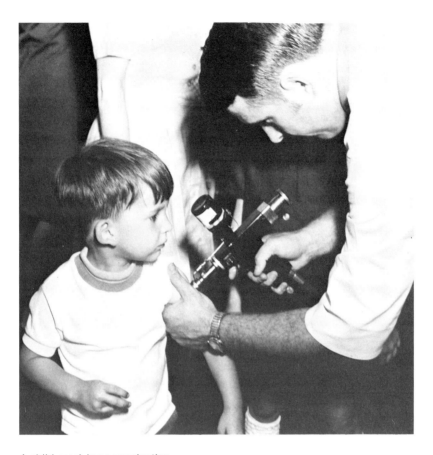

A child receiving a vaccination.

to another. Or they may be produced in animals by injecting them with antigens and then transferred directly to the person. These antibodies are immediately ready for action. This procedure is called *passive immunization* because the person plays no part in actually producing the antibodies. For example, during pregnancy a mother's antibodies pass to her unborn child through the connecting cord that links them.

These antibodies give the baby the same immunities his mother has, and they will last for a short while after birth.

Anyone who has recovered from a disease has some antibodies left over in his system. These antibodies were made to fight this specific disease, and it is possible to take them from this person's body. The antibodies are then injected into a person who has been exposed to the same disease. Thus immunized, the person is usually protected from the disease.

Whether a vaccine substance comes from the blood of an animal or a person, the antibodies are carried in the clear, watery part of the blood known as the *serum*. Any serum used to transfer particular antibodies to someone is called an *antiserum*. Antiserums, if used early enough, can prevent or modify such diseases as measles, diphtheria, poliomyelitis, and tetanus. They can also bolster up the body when it has already been exposed to disease. For example, snake venom antibodies are given after a snakebite. And antianthrax serum is given to a person after exposure to the sheep disease of anthrax.

Passive immunity provides a person with protection for only a few weeks. Active immunization, however, gives much more lasting protection; it may last for years or even for life. Incidentally, the history of a person's immunities is so well "written" into his individual blood that antigens are sometimes used in crime laboratories to tell whether a bloodstain came from one person or another.

It has been known for thousands of years that specific protection against many diseases is conferred by surviv-

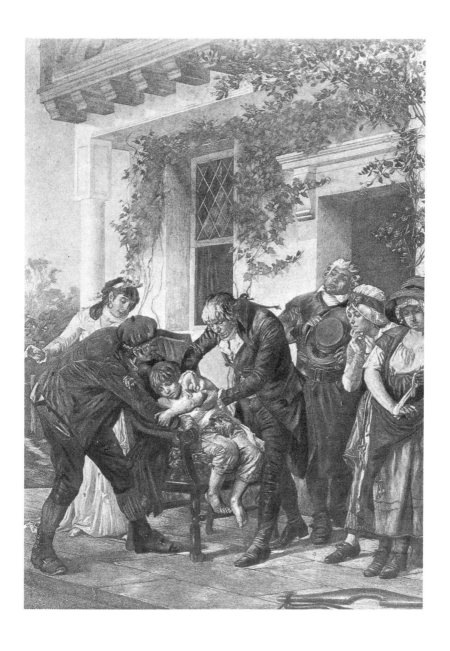

Edward Jenner, English physician, giving his first smallpox vaccination.

ing a first attack of the disease. In practically all the great scourges of history, notably smallpox, yellow fever, bubonic plague, and typhoid fever, someone who was fortunate enough to recover from one illness almost never contracted the same disease again. However, he did remain susceptible to other, unrelated diseases.

Doctors learned to make use of the antibody system of defense long before they knew that such things as antibodies existed. Let us look at some of the milestones in the science of immunology.

A primitive form of immunization against smallpox was practised by the Chinese and Turks in the fifteenth century. In this procedure, scabs from a relatively mild case of smallpox were ground up and inhaled like snuff by persons who had not yet contracted the disease. This practice was believed to ensure protection against the disease, but it probably caused many cases of severe smallpox.

The first serious experiment in immunology was performed by an English country doctor named Edward Jenner. Jenner had observed that milkmaids who had contracted the disease of cowpox never came down later with smallpox, a common killer in Jenner's day. It is now known that the cowpox virus is structurally and chemically related to the smallpox virus, so that immunity to one disease automatically confers immunity to the other. In other words, the antibody elicited by cowpox will also combat the smallpox antigen. But Jenner and other physicians of his time had no way of knowing this. In his famous experiment, Jenner inoculated humans with material from a cowpox sore, producing a mild pustule, or pimplelike blister, in that

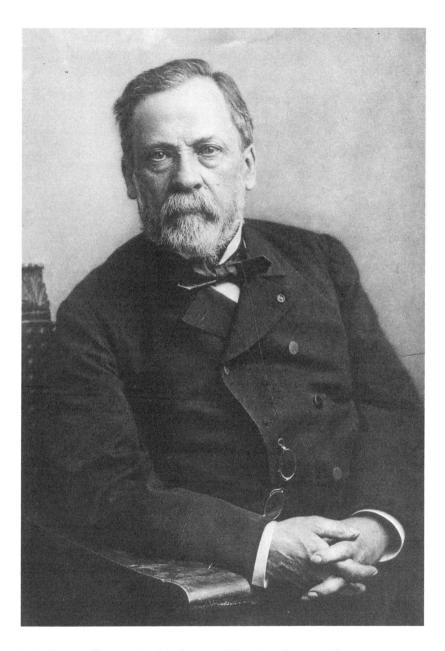

Louis Pasteur, French chemist, discovered that bacteria cause diseases.

area of the skin. He then soon discovered that the people he had inoculated were immune to smallpox.

It was nearly a hundred years before the next step forward was taken in immunology. This advance was the result of the work of the French scientist Louis Pasteur. Pasteur firmly established that putrefaction (decomposition of organic matter) of all sorts, including the formation of pus in the body, depends on the multiplication of living microorganisms. This discovery was rapidly followed by the isolation of a large number of disease-producing microorganisms. One of Pasteur's greatest contributions to science was the development in 1885 of a form of immunization against rabies, a disease carried by dogs and other animals and now known to be caused by viruses. The vaccine Pasteur used is now considered dangerous and not universally effective, but his discovery of the role played by microorganisms in causing infectious diseases laid the foundation for more successful future immunizations.

In 1890, the German scientist Adolph von Behring found that immunity to infectious diseases depends on the presence of certain specific molecules circulating in the bloodstream. It was, in fact, von Behring who gave these molecules their name—antibodies, which in German is *Antikörper*. Working with diphtheria, von Behring found that if one person's antibodies against the toxin produced by diphtheria were injected into another person, they could neutralize diphtheria toxins in the second person. Hence the injected antibodies were called *antitoxins*. The term is still used today and refers to the purified immunizing agent derived from a serum that provides a person with passive immunity.

Since von Behring's time, the science of immunology has moved steadily forward in the conquest of disease. Probably the most dramatic breakthrough in recent history was the discovery by Dr. Jonas Salk of a vaccine against the crippling disease of poliomyelitis. That event is well worth telling here.

Poliomyelitis, also known as infantile paralysis, attacks and destroys the nerve cells and nerve fibers of the human body. It causes fever, cramps, and muscle pains. Since it can destroy the nerve cells connected to muscles, it can also weaken muscles so that they cannot function.

At the beginning of 1955, polio was the leading cause of physical handicaps in young children. One-fifth of the crippled people in the United States were polio victims. In 1952, the United States' worst epidemic—about 58,000 cases—resulted in some 3,000 deaths. Up to that time, the National Foundation for Infantile Paralysis and groups of scientists had worked for many years to find some way of controlling this dread disease.

Earlier, in 1909, it had been learned that polio is caused by a virus germ. Later it was shown that there are actually three distinct types of polio viruses, each of which produces a different variety of the disease. In 1949, a group of Harvard scientists grew polio virus in test tubes containing monkey kidney tissue. This made it possible to get a readily available supply of the virus for a possible vaccine.

Other scientists had demonstrated that the polio virus traveled in the bloodstream before it reached and

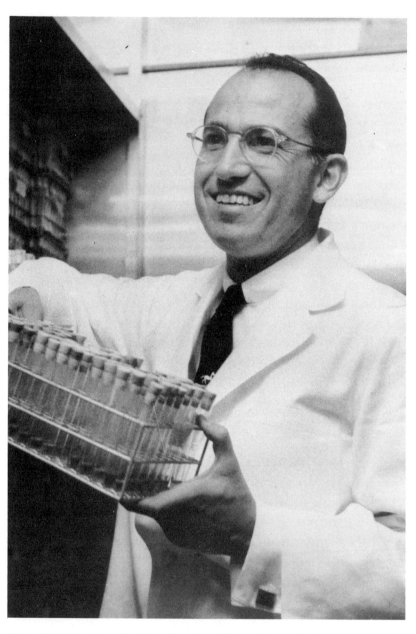

Jonas Salk, American physician, inventor of the polio vaccination.

58

destroyed the nerve centers. Could a vaccine be developed that could build up defensive antibodies in the blood to combat the polio virus?

In 1950, Dr. Jonas Salk, a thirty-five-year-old scientist at the University of Pittsburgh, was given money by the National Foundation for Infantile Paralysis to fight the polio virus. Salk's idea was to develop a vaccine from dead viruses. By 1951, he had made a series of experimental vaccines and had tested them on monkeys. In 1952, he was sure enough of his vaccine to try it out on his own children. There were no ill effects when he did so.

In the spring of 1954, the National Foundation decided to test the Salk vaccine and set up the greatest medical experiment ever undertaken. A total of 422,743 children in forty-four states were given the vaccine. As a control group, about an equal number of children were given "dummy" injections of harmless material. About the same number who received no shots at all were also observed in the experiment. During the summer and fall of 1954, scientists collected data from all these children in the experiment. It was a tremendous undertaking to collect all this information and subject it to study.

Finally, on April 12, 1955, the results of this triumph of the scientific method were announced to the world: "The Salk vaccine works. It is safe, effective, and potent."

Since that time, millions of children have been vaccinated against polio with the Salk vaccine. As yet, it does not provide 100 percent protection; a small number of children did not become immune. But it has been

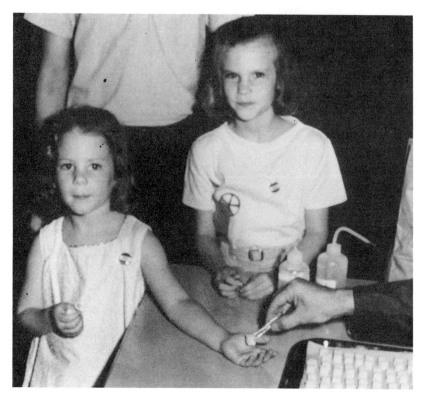

Children receiving the Sabin vaccine.

effective in the vast majority of cases and the total conquest of polio is well on its way. Moreover, a newer antipolio vaccine, called the Sabin vaccine after its discoverer, has been enlisted in the fight against the ravages of polio. Unlike the Salk vaccine, it is not given by injection but by mouth. The Sabin vaccine contains live viruses instead of dead ones. You yourself have probably had one or more of these vaccines in recent years.

The science of immunology today is much concerned

with two other human afflictions against which the body must defend itself. One, allergy, is more of a constant nuisance to the sufferer than it is potentially fatal. The other, the dread disease of cancer in its several forms, is presently immunology's Public Enemy Number One. Oddly, the two are related in the sense that they both represent a kind of immunological backfiring, or "double cross." That is, sometimes the vital human defense system attacks and harms the body's own tissues—the very tissues it is supposed to defend.

Allergies are abnormal overresponses, to certain substances which may cause asthma, hay fever, and other allergic diseases. When an antigen and an antibody unite on the surface of certain cells, this union can trigger the release of special biochemical agents stored in the cell. Such agents include the two complex chemical compounds histamine and serotonin, both of which have powerful effects on the blood vessels and the muscles. When kept within bounds, these reactions can help the body's defense system, but if excessive, they can do serious harm. The actual function of histamine and serotonin in the body is not presently known.

Some of the most common forms of allergy are eczema, hay fever, and various food allergies. Allergic reactions from the stings of bees, wasps, hornets, and other insects are also common. The antigens involved are known as *allergens.* Some allergens that trigger familiar allergic symptoms like hives, itching, sneezing, cramps, and nausea are plant pollens, household dust, feathers, ragweed, certain dyes and metals, nail polish, skin medications, dog and cat hair, and various foods such as strawberries and shellfish.

Allergens usually enter the body through some natural point of entry, such as the digestive tract or respiratory system. About ten percent of all people have an inborn tendency to form excessive amounts of antibodies against allergens. Research in allergy is now seriously directed toward the question of how this overproduction of antibodies can be controlled and kept in reasonable check. This research is supported by various government, private, and philanthropic agencies, all of whom are eager to put an end to these irritating human miseries.

For reasons not yet fully understood by medical science, certain cells in the body may suddenly undergo abnormal changes and begin to reproduce at an unusual rate. This uncontrolled, irregular cell growth is called *cancer*. Instead of dividing in two as is normal, a cancerous cell may split to form three, four, or more new cells. The cells become irregular in size and shape. They do not stop multiplying. The nucleus, or inner center, of the cancer cell shows the most dramatic signs of abnormality, appearing larger than normal and distorted in shape. Masses of these abnormal cells eventually form a lump or swelling which is called a *tumor*.

There are actually two main classes of tumors—benign and malignant. *Benign*—meaning "mild" or "gentle"—tumors are made up of cells which tend to differ only slightly from normal cells or tissues. Benign tumors do not generally endanger life since the cells in them do not invade other areas of the body. If, however, a cancerous cell growth penetrates surrounding areas and spreads, it is a *malignant* (meaning "death-threatening") tumor. Unless it is destroyed or removed, a

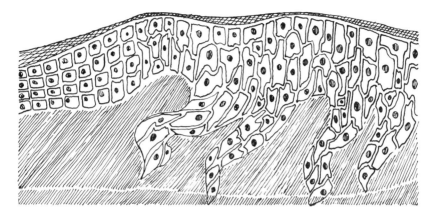

A diagram showing how a malignant cancer tumor looks.

malignant tumor may cause a person's death. The abnormal cells may also break off and enter the bloodstream or lymph channels and be carried to other parts of the body, where they establish deadly new colonies.

Over 200 different kinds of cancer are presently recognized in man. The disease can occur in any organ of the body; however, it is most commonly found in the breast (male or female), the stomach, the colon (large intestine), the skin, the lungs, and the uterus. Less common is cancerous growth in the liver, throat, lungs, bone, testes, and pancreas.

Many scientists now believe that cancer cells succeed in growing and spreading because of a failure on the part of the immunity system to recognize and attack them. In laboratory animals, it has been shown that most cancerous cells are chemically different from the other body cells: the cancer cells carry antigens. Usually, however, they are rather weak antigens, and it is probably because of their weakness that the immunity mechanisms of the animal cannot be sufficently aroused to reject the cancerous tumor growth. Although there is a battle between the growing tumor and the animal's lymphocytes, the cancer eventually wins.

Working with laboratory animals, medical scientists have discovered ways to make the immune response to the antigens in cancer cells so strong that the tumor *is* rejected. Today, a large branch of active research is concerned with tumor behavior. Even so, scientists have not yet been able to develop a method of immunotherapy or an immune protective against cancer. But if, as is widely supposed by medical scientists, tumors get out of hand because of some fault on the part of the body's protective machinery, then understanding immunity recognition and what makes it go wrong should lead to more effective ways of treating one of mankind's most deadly disorders.

Although sometimes the human immunity system cannot do enough of a job—as in the case of cancer—at other times it does its job all too well, as in the case of organ transplant rejection. Specifically, the body recognizes a new heart, a new kidney, a new liver as something "nonself"—as something strange and completely foreign. Thus our marvelous—and relentless—immunity mechanism once again gears up its antibodies for the search-and-destroy mission that will reject the new organ. The fact that so many times the immunity system will not allow such transplants to "take" is one of modern biology's greatest ironies.

In any discussion of immunology, *autoimmune diseases* must also be mentioned. These diseases are supposed to be caused by the body's developing an immune reaction to some of its own tissues and cells, as if they

64

were infectious organisms. The processes by which an autoimmune condition may arise have not yet been fully explained. Somehow, perhaps as a reaction to shock or injury or as a result of heredity, antibodies attack the tissues of certain organs or even of the entire body instead of directing their attacks to invading organisms. They produce inflammation, breakdown, and even degeneration of the parts that are affected.

Among the diseases that are strongly suspected of being of autoimmune origin are rheumatoid arthritis, which cripples joints; lupus erythematosus, involving the entire body and especially the connective tissue; multiple sclerosis, a disease of the nervous system; myasthenia gravis, a disease that attacks the muscles; and hemolytic anemia, an affliction that destroys the blood cells.

In recent years, the tempo of research in immunology has quickened dramatically. As a result, the immunity system has been coaxed to yield more and more of its secrets. Yet many important questions about the body's defense machinery still remain. Among them is: How does the human body really detect the presence of hostile invaders? One world-famous biologist, who is hard at work on the mystery, put it this way: "This riddle of recognition is one of the burning issues of modern biology."

· 7 ·

When the Body
Recovers From Disease and Injury

·

Other Defenses of the Body

A few infections are so massive or violent that they swiftly overwhelm all local and secondary resistance and enter the bloodstream. In some instances, deadly microbes are introduced directly into the blood itself. These disorders are known as *general infections*. Unless previous immunization has been given, they are often serious and sometimes fatal.

Two examples of general infections are typhoid fever and the blood poisoning known as septicemia.

General infections may be overcome by the human body's own immunity mechanism through the gradual development of antibodies. The progress of the disease indicates the struggle between the body's defenses and the invading antigens. What are the possible outcomes? Either the result is victory (recovery); defeat (death); or a stalemate (chronic, or continuing, disease).

Assuming that the body's defenses are victorious, what happens when the body recovers from disease or injury?

When the body's forces have been mobilized for defense and have won the action, the local site of the skirmish begins to clear up. The healing processes take place and, if the skin has been broken, a scar often remains. Once they have gone into action, however, the body defenses remain on the alert for further trouble. The tissues that have reacted against an invasion by a communicable disease do not stop reacting when the emergency has passed. They go on producing the defensive substances which continue to circulate in the blood.

For example, the blood of a person who has recovered from typhoid fever contains agglutinins, which cause living typhoid bacteria to cluster together. The presence of such antibodies gives a person protection which wears out only after a period of years. That is why second cases of communicable diseases are rare; people who do suffer such diseases a second time have weakened powers of defense and may become more seriously ill than a normal person, or they may even die.

Even after a person has recovered from disease, injury, or surgery, certain organs or tissues may have been more or less seriously damaged. In these cases, the body may go on functioning quite well, but only as long as there are no unusual stresses upon it. Before the days of modern drug treatment, for example, scarlet fever often did serious damage to the kidneys, destroying some cells and damaging others. In some instances, recovery would take place under proper treatment. If the injury to the cells had not been too great, they would recover and assume their function. Those cells which had been killed would be partially replaced by other cells of similar character or by fibrous scar tissue.

If in the healing process after injury, disease, or surgical removal, too much scar tissue is left and too few cells are replaced, the patient is limited in the ways he can function. Why? Because scar tissue that is left after injury to, say, the skin consists of specialized fibrous tissue and does not represent actual replacement of the original cells. The scar tissue lacks elasticity and the epidermis is not attached firmly to it.

Even so, the body has a final line of defense against such limitation of function. In many cases, there is so much reserve tissue that there will be enough of it to meet the ordinary needs of the body. Hence, many people with injured tissues or organs can live normal lives by taking good care of themselves and following the instructions of their doctors.

After injury, many of the body's tissues can be, and are, replaced. Skin, muscles, and even bone are capable of healing well and full function is restored, except in very severe cases. The mucous membranes of the stomach, lungs, intestines, and other internal organs are still able to carry on after they have suffered extensive injury. In the liver and kidneys, there is much more substance than is required for normal living; if some is lost, more of the reserve is called upon. Vital organs such as the heart have a high rate of recovery after serious injury due to diphtheria, rheumatic fever, or even a heart attack.

How are our bodies able to renew themselves in these ways? This is one of the functions of *metabolism*, which refers to all the chemical reactions in living tissue, particularly in the production of energy, the manufacture of tissue, and the formation of waste products. Metabolism is one of the attributes of life; when an organism dies, metabolism ceases. During life, energy production and the manufacture of new and rejuvenating tissue are made possible by the chemical nutrients in the food we eat. Perhaps you have heard doctors talk about the *basal metabolic rate*. This is the rate at which a person expends energy to maintain the life processes while he is awake, at rest, and not eating or drinking. Doctors can measure the expended energy in terms of how much heat the body produces, usually determined by the amount of oxygen consumed and carbon dioxide eliminated in a definite time period.

Certain organs of the body may, to some extent, even take over the functions of others that have been put out of commission. For example, the stomach can be almost completely removed and digestion still go on in the intestines with hardly diminished efficiency, provided a few eating habits are changed. Failure or removal of glands can now be remedied by supplying the body with the hormones they would normally produce. Two examples are taking thyroid tablets by mouth and replacing insulin by injection.

Unfortunately, once they have been destroyed, some specialized tissues are not replaceable by healing. For example, vision is permanently lost when the optic nerve which leads to the eye, is destroyed. Likewise, when the nerve of hearing is gone, that faculty is lost forever.

Similarly, when the cells of special sense nerves and of the brain and spinal cord are killed, they are not replaced by other nerve cells but by scar tissue. Thus when a brain area concerned with a certain function, such as the muscle control of a hand or foot, is destroyed, the hand or foot will be paralyzed unless other muscles can take the place of the lost muscle. While it is true that sometimes recovery, or at least partial recovery, may occur after a brain injury, this is because the nerve cells have not been destroyed but only injured. As they recover, their function returns.

Many nerve cells have long filaments carrying impulses to a distant point or bringing them from that point. If such a filament is cut but the cell remains intact, function will return when a new filament has grown along the path of the injured one.

When the healing process involves less specialized tissues, new cells are formed only to the extent that the tissue is made whole again and resumes its function. In a normal person, regrowth and scarring after an injury or surgery seldom get out of control. In a few cases, a

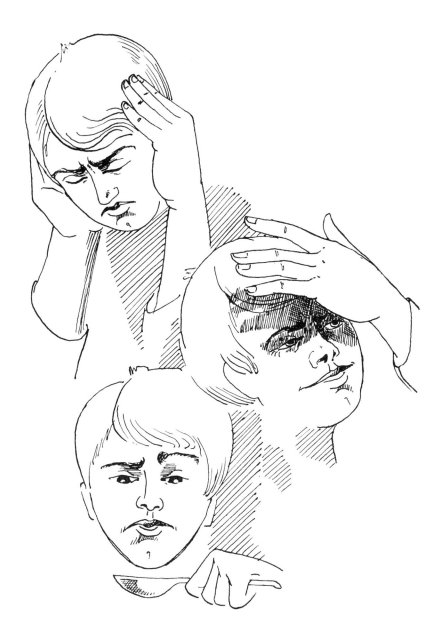

Psychological defenses to loud noise, bright sunlight and noticing something repellent in food.

scar may be overgrown to form a structure known as a keloid, which can usually be corrected by minor surgery.

In addition to all the human defenses we have already considered, there are still others which serve us daily. These are our psychological and mental defenses, arising out of instinctive fears and the experience we build up as we go through life. We are born, for example, with the innate fear of falling and loud noises. Thus we instinctively avoid dangerously high places, a fall from which would injure our bodies. And we clap our hands automatically over our ears when excessive noise threatens injury to the nerve of hearing.

As we grow older and hopefully wiser, we develop by experience various patterns of cautious behavior to keep us out of trouble and reasonably safe most of the time. We learn how to drive defensively in our automobiles to avoid tragedy on the expressways. At sea, we observe safety rules to keep our craft intact and afloat and ourselves from drowning. In the home, we learn how to handle fire and electricity so that they will not harm us but serve us. We form the habit of dressing warmly and sensibly so that our resistance does not become lowered, paving the way for invading cold viruses.

But even when our mental and psychological faculties fail us and we become injured or diseased, we are sure of one thing: the body's amazing protective machinery is ready to go into action the minute it is needed. For the survival of mankind itself depends on the smooth meshing of this marvelous and complex machinery.

·Appendix·
Good Health
and Your Body's Defenses
·
Some Basic Guidelines

Although your body's defenses are ready to go into action the minute danger threatens, it stands to reason that the better physical shape you are in, the better they can serve you. Obviously, if your general resistance is low or you have let yourself become run down in any way, your defenses

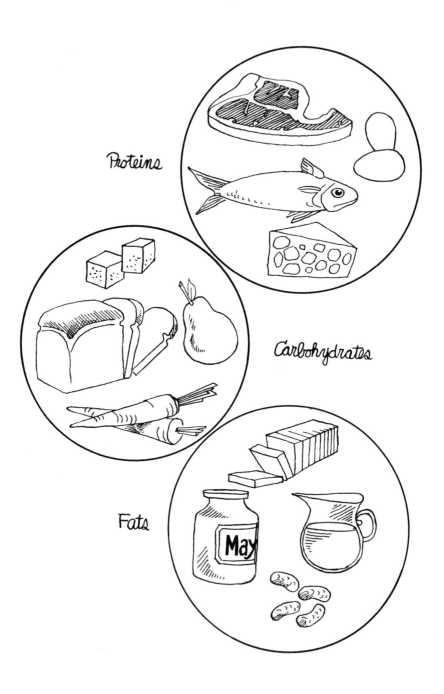

Proteins

Carbohydrates

Fats

74

will have to work doubly hard to overcome invading infections. Therefore, a brief review of some guidelines to good health is in order for all readers of this book.

When your body is well, your mind is sound and active, and you feel in good spirits, you are in good health. Body, mind, and emotions are closely related, and the well-being of all three is essential to good health. But keeping the body well is the foundation of good health. The best way to keep your body strong and sound is to see that it is cared for properly.

Proper care of your body begins with a good diet. The foods you eat and the liquids you drink supply the body with the materials it needs to do its work and grow.

Different foods contain different substances needed by your body. Foods like milk, meat, cheese, eggs, and fish contain proteins. These are substances needed to repair and build muscle and bone. Proteins also supply some of the fuel that the body turns into energy. Carbohydrates and fats are the body's main sources of energy. Foods like bread, cereals, fruits, vegetables, and sugar contain carbohydrates. Butter, mayonnaise, nuts, and cream contain fats.

If your diet includes proteins, fats, and carbohydrates, it also includes the vitamins and minerals you need. Vitamins are chemicals that help your body make proper use of the food you eat daily. Minerals help build some of the body's structures and aid in adjusting some of its functions. In certain cases—perhaps your own—a doctor may feel that extra vitamins are necessary, and he will recommend them.

Your body also needs water. It is needed to help carry food to the cells and to aid in getting rid of waste material. Since most foods contain water, a large part of your daily need is provided by the foods you eat. In addition, however, you should drink several glasses of liquid each day.

The food you eat supplies your body with energy; this energy is measured in units of heat called *calories*. The number of calories you need each day depends upon the amount of energy your body requires. Different people have different energy needs, depending on their size, the rate at which they are growing, and their activities. If you are a boy or girl from twelve to eighteen years of age, you are going through your period of greatest growth right now. At this time your calory needs are high.

If you gain weight at a normal rate during this period of your life, you know that you are supplying your body with the right number of calories for growth and activity. If you are putting on more weight than is normal, you are supplying your body with more energy than it is using up. The extra food is being turned into fat and stored up by your body.

If, on the other hand, you tend to lose weight, you are probably not eating enough to supply your body with the energy it needs. Your body is drawing on its reserve supplies of fat to make up for the calories it is not receiving.

With the help of your physician, you can decide whether your present weight is right for you. If it turns out that you would be better off losing weight, it will help to follow two principles: get as much exercise as you can in order to burn up extra food energy and be careful about eating the "fuel foods" (fats, starches, and sweets). Stick to fish, lean meats, vegetables, and fruits. But, don't try to diet by skipping meals. Your energy supply will be lowered when you go without food for long stretches, and you won't be able to do your most productive work.

If you are underweight, you can gain by adding carbohydrates and fats to your diet. Especially important are fats because they provide twice as much energy, or calories, as carbohydrates.

In each twenty-four-hour period, your body requires a number of hours of absolute rest during which its functions slow down. While medical science has not yet found out all the changes that take place in the body during sleep, it is generally agreed that this is the time in which the cells recover from the work of the daytime and build up new supplies of energy for the next day. Most doctors recommend that boys and girls of elementary and high school ages have from eight to ten hours of sleep each night.

One of the most important parts of the daily care of your body is exercise. This physical activity helps keep weight under control by using some of the energy supplied by food. Exercise is good for the blood vessels because it helps keep even the smaller ones—the capillaries—open. Daily exercise also keeps your muscles toned up and healthy.

Daily exercise means just that. You should set aside a definite amount of time each day for exercise—but the choice is up to you. You can swim, walk, skate, dance, ride your bike, lift weights, do calisthenics, or play tennis, baseball, football, or basketball. The point is: Keep your blood circulation moving.

While a balanced diet, exercise, and enough sleep are all necessary for your general health, the right kind of care is also necessary for the health of particular parts of your body.

THE SKIN. The main rule to follow in caring for the skin is to keep it clean. Through the small openings in the skin called pores, oil and sweat pass from the glands onto the surface of the skin. Dirt also collects on the skin. By washing with soap and water, you prevent sweat, oil, and dirt from blocking the pores and causing pimples and blackheads. You also help remove germs that may cause infections or boils. Make a habit of taking a bath or shower once a day, and always wash your hands before eating and after going to the bathroom.

To prevent infection on the skin of your hands and feet, follow these rules. Never cut the cuticle or skin at the base and sides of the nails; press it back gently with an orange stick. Always cut hangnails; never try to bite or pull them off. Cracks, redness, and itching of the skin between and around the toes may be signs of athlete's foot, a fungus infection. This condition should be seen and treated by your doctor. Blisters and calluses on the skin of your feet may mean that your shoes have not been properly fitted.

THE HAIR. The blood that flows to the scalp nourishes the roots of your hair. When you brush your hair, you increase the supply of blood to the scalp. That is why daily brushing is good for the hair. Normal hair should be shampooed at least once a week. If your hair is oily, you may shampoo two or more times a week. If it's dry, you may prefer to wash it once every two weeks.

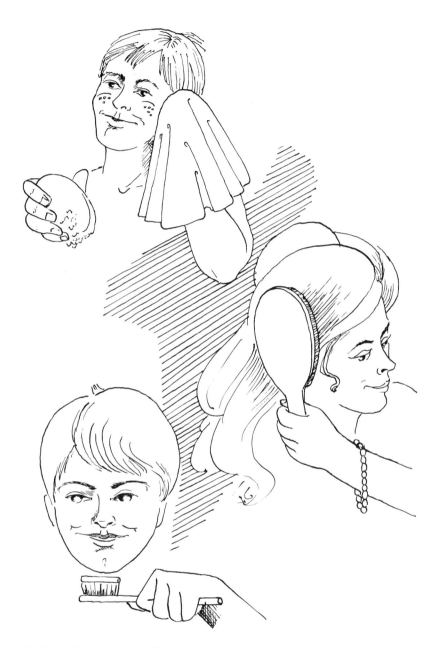

Health habits: washing, hair care and dental care.

79

THE EYES. Never rub your eyes. You may scratch the part of the eye through which you see (the cornea). If you feel there is something in your eye, if it is red, if you have a sty (an infection of the lid), or if you have injured your eye, don't try to treat it yourself with eyewashes or drops. See a doctor. Also, never stare at a source of ultraviolet light, such as the sun, a sunlamp, or an acetylene torch, or you may permanently damage your eyes.

THE EARS. The outer parts of the ears should be washed when you bathe or shower. It is normal for earwax to form in the canal leading from the outer to the inner ear, but do not attempt to clean out this wax yourself. With most people, excess wax will simply fall out of the ear in a ball from time to time. Never put an object of any kind in your ear canal. You may injure the eardrum. If wax collects and blocks the canal, it should be cleaned out by a physician. An earache or any difficulty in hearing should be reported to your doctor.

THE TEETH. To keep your teeth and gums healthy, it is necessary to have a balanced diet. You should also do all you can to prevent tooth decay. This means brushing your teeth well after meals and avoiding between-meal soft drinks, candy, and other sweets. If sugar is left in your mouth after eating, harmful bacteria can act on the sugar to form an acid. This acid can eat into the hard outer covering (enamel) of your teeth and cause a cavity. In any case, form the habit of seeing your dentist once every six months for a checkup.

YOUR DOCTOR CAN HELP. Be sure to call your doctor if you have an illness or fever of any kind. When you are ill, follow his advice about caring for yourself. Tell

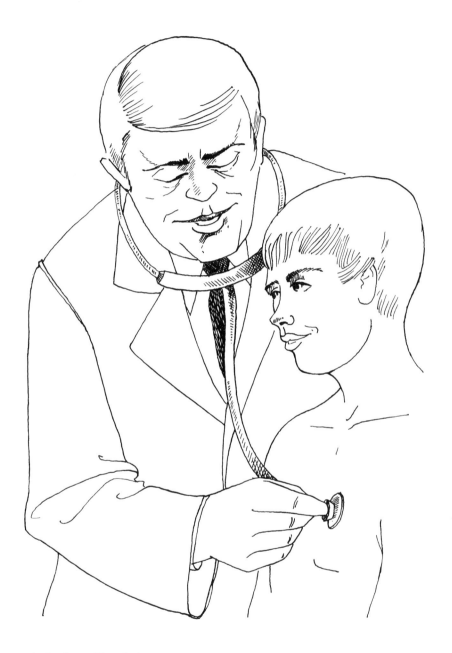

A checkup with a doctor.

him right away if you are bothered by sore throats, nosebleeds, headaches, earaches, or other discomforts. Even if you feel in good health, make it a point to have him check you over at least once a year. He will examine you and make sure that you are protected against tetanus, diphtheria, polio, measles, and whooping cough.

COMMON SENSE IN AVOIDING DANGERS. One of the greatest threats to the health of boys and girls in their school years is accidents. You can help prevent them by obeying traffic, water safety, and fire prevention rules.

Certain habits are to be avoided, too. Soon you may begin to think about smoking. While this habit was once considered relatively harmless, many physicians and scientists now believe that smoking is really quite harmful to the blood vessels and lungs. Thus, they are urging that young people not start the habit.

You should also avoid taking medicines and drugs on your own. They may be harmful to you, and taking them may cover up a problem that needs a doctor's attention. A good common-sense rule to follow is to never take medicine of any kind unless a physician orders it and instructs you in how much to take. In addition, avoid treating yourself with laxatives, vitamins, cold medicines, pills to kill pain, stay-awake or sleeping pills, or weight reducers.

Although protecting and guarding your health is a lifetime job, it is a job that is worth doing well. Good health makes it possible for you to participate fully in all that goes on around you and to live each day with enjoyment. But if something does go wrong, good health will also guarantee that your body's defenses will spring into action with maximum effectiveness.

82

Glossary

Glossary

Abscess   A collection of pus in the body; a boil.

Acquired immunity   Resistance to an invading organism that a person develops himself through production of antibodies. Also called artificial immunity.

Active immunization   Procedure whereby a vaccinated person makes his own antibodies against disease rather than getting them from someone else.

Allergen   An antigen that produces an allergy.

Allergy   Abnormal overresponse to certain substances which results in such allergic diseases as hay fever or asthma.

Amino acids Nitrogen-containing chemical substances that constitute the building blocks from which plant and animal tissues are made. The proteins found in all living things are composed of amino acids.

Antibodies Protein molecules produced within the body to counteract the effects of invading antigens.

Antigens Complex invading chemicals which, when recognized by the body, stimulate the production of antibodies. Microorganisms which can serve as antigens include bacteria, protozoa, molds, yeasts and viruses.

Antiserum Any serum used to transfer antibodies from one person (or animal) to another.

Antitoxins Antibodies formed in the body as a result of the introduction of a toxin, capable of neutralizing the specific toxin which stimulated their production.

Autoimmune disease Any disease presumed to be caused by the body's developing an immune reaction to some of its own tissues and cells, as if they were infectious organisms.

Bacteria Microscopic one-celled plants, some of which are capable of causing disease.

Capillaries Slender hairlike tubes that are the smallest vessels in the blood-carrying system of the body.

Cell A small mass of the living substance that is the basis of all plant and animal life, with its surrounding walls.

Dermis The layer of skin directly under the outer layer or epidermis; also called the "true skin."

Epidermis The outer layer of skin covering the human body.

General infection An infection so massive or violent that it overwhelms the body's defenses and enters the bloodstream.

Germ A microorganism that causes disease.

Globulins A group of proteins to which antibodies belong.

Hemorrhage An excessive loss of blood.

Hormone A complex organic compound which controls cell metabolism and growth.

Immune response The reaction of the human body in getting rid of—or attempting to get rid of—invading antigens.

Immunology The scientific study of how the human body resists invasion by outside substances.

Infection Any disease caused by germs.

Inflammation process A local response to cellular injury

86

marked by swelling, redness, heat, and usually the formation of pus. It serves as a mechanism initialing elimination of infectious material and the repair of damaged tissue.

Inoculate   To give a disease to a person or animal in a mild form in order to prevent any other attack.

Lymph nodes   Collections of spongy tissue in the body which constitute strainer-like traps for infectious germs.

Lymphocytes   White cells in the body which encourage the formation of antibodies.

Melanin   A pigment contained in the epidermis.

Metabolism   All the chemical processes in a living organism that convert food and oxygen into tissues and energy.

Microbe   A germ; a plant or animal so small that it can be seen only through a microscope. The term is usually applied to a microorganism of an infectious nature.

Microorganism   A tiny living plant or animal that can only be seen under a microscope; a microbe or a germ. Some are harmful to man but most are harmless.

Molds   Usually harmless, threadlike plants which grow on food. Some can grow on human skin and can cause disease.

Mucous membrane   Tissue lining the mouth, nose, alimentary canal and body openings that is waterproof and resists invasion by germs.

Native immunity   The resistance the human body has at birth to many different invading organisms.

Pain   A feeling of discomfort or distress arising from disease, injury, or bodily disorder.

Passive immunization   A type of immunity in which a person plays no part in actually producing antibodies. Such antibodies may be taken from one person and given to another by injection or inoculation, or transferred from a mother to her child during pregnancy.

Phagocytes   White blood cells that are active in surrounding and destroying unwanted germs in the body.

Physiology   The science that studies the functions of the parts of the human body, such as organs, tissues and cells.

Proteins   Large groups of complex nourishing compounds found in all living plant and animal cells, and made up of over 20 amino acids. A necessary element in diet, supplied by such foods as meat, milk, or eggs.

Protozoa Tiny one-celled animals, most of which are microscopic. Very few cause human disease, but some are very harmful, such as the protozoan that causes malaria.

Pus The fluid that gathers in abscesses as a reaction to inflammation caused by germs. It consists mainly of white blood cells, dead tissue cells, and living or dead germs.

Reflex action An involuntary response performed as a consequence of a nervous impulse transmitted inward from a sensory receptor to a nerve center and outward again to a muscle or gland—the whole process culminating in an act such as ducking or withdrawing one's hand from a hot fire.

Sensory receptors Sensitive cells or groups of cells located near the surface of the skin, capable of conveying nerve impulses to nerve centers.

Serum The watery part of the blood separated from the solid part; especially such a fluid obtained from the blood and used as an antitoxin to prevent or cure disease.

Subcutaneous fat A fatty layer of tissue beneath the dermis.

Tissue A mass of cells, together with the substance containing them, from which the human body is built up; such as muscular tissue.

Toxin A poison, produced by an animal, a plant, or germs; as, a snake toxin, or the toxin of diphtheria germs.

Tumor An abnormal or diseased mass of tissue arising without obvious cause from cells of pre-existent tissue and serving no useful purpose. Benign when localized and harmless; malignant if diseased and spreads to other parts of the body.

Vaccination The act of producing immunity in a person by either injecting or orally taking vaccine to prevent a serious attack of a specific disease.

Vaccine The substance made from germs which is taken orally or injected into the body in vaccination.

Viruses Any of several simple disease-causing microorganisms smaller than bacteria.

Yeasts Microscopic single-celled living plants, most of which are harmless. A few are harmful to man.

Index

Index

92

94